I0436541

Seven Movements to Keep you Gardening for Life

Dan Tatton & John Sinclair

DEDICATION

I would like to dedicate this book to my Bauba. Some of my favorite childhood memories involve spending time in the garden with you. As one of the most selfless and giving people I have ever known you inspired this book that's main purpose is to help others.
— Dan Tatton

CONTENTS

ACKNOWLEDGMENTS

A special thank you goes out to Jennifer Tatton for providing her editing services for this book and Marie–Lise Norris for the cover design.

Also a special thank you to Patricia Sullivan who graciously invited us into her garden and posed as our model for the movement section of this book.

WHY YOU NEED THIS BOOK

Whether you're an avid gardener or someone who does a little gardening here and there, this book will change your life forever. We can change your perspective on what you consider exercise to be for you. By connecting exercise to an activity you love doing, you will find that we have developed an exercise program for gardeners that will build strength around the most common movements and positions of your craft. We want to make your exercise relevant to your needs.

Getting older does not mean you should have to endure more pain and it is never too late to start moving. We are going to teach you how an investment of seven minutes of your day can change your life and keep you gardening on your terms. We will show you how to connect with your exercise and give it purpose. By integrating the information and activities provided in this book into your daily life, you will develop the habits to strengthen and prepare the body for the gardening you love.

Exercise is more enjoyable when it is centered around something we love to do and we see exercise less as a chore and more as a way of life that energizes us and sustains us.

1 THINK

Changing the paradigm

We want to change the way you look at exercise. The human mind, body, and spirit crave movement just to survive and, when we keep it simple, we find the most consistent results. Unfortunately many people today feel like the only way to experience movement is to spend endless hours in the gym. This creates a dichotomy of either exercising excessively or not at all. Most people choose the latter since the former is too unrealistic and we get convinced that a small amount of exercise just isn't worth it. The result is we are not exercising enough, sedentary diseases are on the rise, and people are spending the final years of their lives in wheelchairs or bedridden. We must alter our attitude towards exercise in a very fundamental way. But before we delve into why giving us seven minutes for seven movements can change your life forever we need to examine our current paradigm as it pertains to how we think and feel about exercise.

Our Current Paradigm

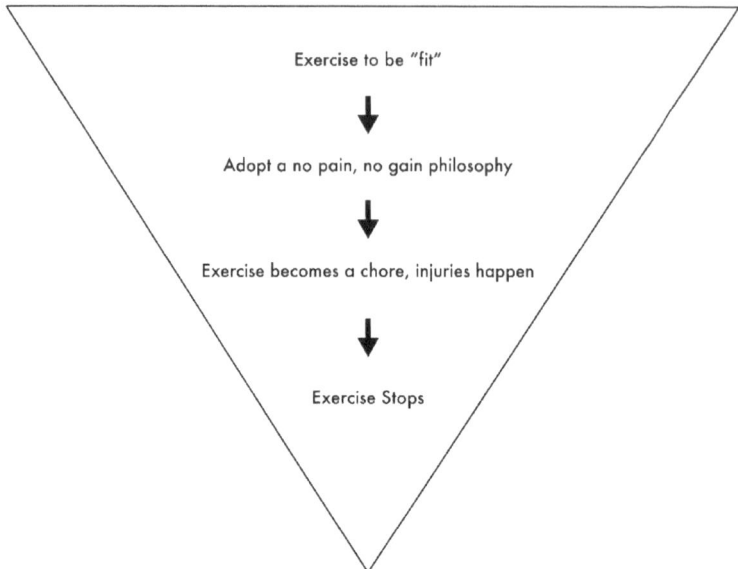

Exercise to be "fit"

↓

Adopt a no pain, no gain philosophy

↓

Exercise becomes a chore, injuries happen

↓

Exercise Stops

When we ask our average client about why he or she started an exercise program we generally get one of two answers: to lose weight or to "get fit". The second question we ask is what comes to mind when you hear the word "exercise"? And the same three words always come up: work, pain, and sweat. Now these are hardly words that would inspire a person to jump on the exercise program bandwagon. As personal trainers, we have watched countless people with the goal of "getting fit" make it a chore to go to the gym because they feel exercise needs to be difficult to be effective. These people will spend countless hours in the gym staring at themselves in the thousands of mirrors to dwell on every tiny flaw in their body. Millions of people join gyms in January and stick with their program until March before quitting more miserable, tired, and defeated than they started out. These people have bought into the message that in order to succeed they must "push through the pain" and never give up. This type of message is not only unrealistic, but can lead to injury later on.

How did this happen? How did we turn something as beautiful and necessary as movement into something we would rather not do? It started with advertising through the mainstream fitness industry that gave us such slogans as "no pain, no gain", that told people if they were not experiencing pain they were not working hard enough. To our dismay, this is still a strongly held belief amongst many who call themselves fitness professionals today. The way this image of exercise affects our psyche today is obvious. We have TV shows with screaming "personal trainers" belittling those to work so hard they feel pain. People running on treadmills in so much pain they cannot even stand up straight, and worse yet, they are not even going anywhere! This type of exercise is not functional but fashionable. This attitude is not only wrong but it will affect your ability to experience any movement in a positive way. So it is no surprise that when we say the word exercise most people immediately associate it with something they *have* to do rather than something they *want* to do.

There is nothing more tragic than watching someone have to stop doing something they love because it now causes them pain. Most people don't realize they are not moving correctly until they start feeling pain, they are then told that pain equals progress. However, this pain generally lands them in the doctor's office where they are given a magic pill and told to get to the gym and start exercising. And the cycle continues. When I see a gardener pulling out weeds and tending to plants I see someone lunging, pulling, and twisting. All incredibly important movements that are, in fact, exercises but, for some reason, we do not call them that. When is the last time you heard someone say they were going to the garden after work to exercise? We need to change this attitude as soon as we can.

The New Seven Movements Paradigm

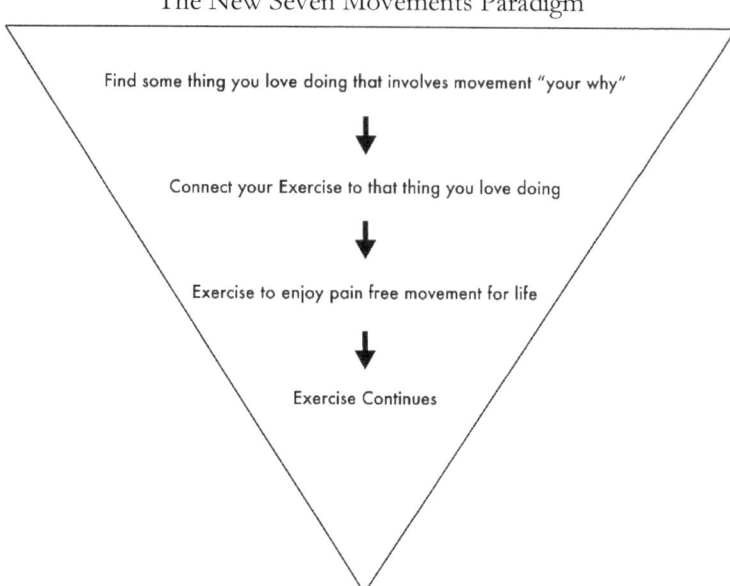

Find some thing you love doing that involves movement "your why"

Connect your Exercise to that thing you love doing

Exercise to enjoy pain free movement for life

Exercise Continues

In our new paradigm we look at exercise in a completely different way. We are going to allow gardening to become our exercise and give our strength training program purpose. We will allow our exercise to compliment the common movements and positions of a gardener. Our ancestors took care of their movement through everyday living. Modern convenience has changed this and in some ways it is a good thing; in other ways, not so much. We have been given the gift of being able to enjoy movement doing the things we love. Our exercise programs can be functional and efficient and this book gives you a program that will allow you to eliminate pain, reduce injury, build strength, and continue pursuing your craft for years to come. Give us seven minutes and we will keep you gardening for life reaping all the rewards of regular exercise not to mention the joy of growing beautiful flowers and delicious food.

When you give exercise purpose you will not only view exercise in a positive light but you will be astonished at the progress you make. You will begin to wonder how it is you are losing weight, having more energy, and getting stronger. Exercise will no longer be work, it will be the expression of movement it is meant to be. You will also be getting stronger with the movements and positions common to gardening meaning you will reduce your chance of injury and eliminate pain from incorrect movement doing repetitive tasks. Pain and weakness will never be the reason you stop gardening, the goal of this book is to keep you gardening for life.

Finding your *Why*: Reconnecting to Movement

When we start a new exercise program with someone we ask them to tell us their *why*. What is their purpose for wanting to exercise? Finding your *why* allows you to connect with your movement and it becomes much more than just exercise. It gives your exercise purpose beyond "getting fit" and allows you to connect with your true goals.

Finding your why is simple. Just ask yourself: What is it I love doing that involves movement? This will allow you to connect instantly to why it is you love moving in the first place. Do you enjoy playing with your kids or grandkids? Kayaking? Do you enjoy golfing without back pain? Is it the reward of a beautiful garden filled with fresh produce and lush flowers? Being fit is nothing more than a symptom of finding your *why* and applying the principles in this book. When you connect exercise to gardening it will affect your entire attitude towards exercise. Exercise is about learning to move, connecting with your body, and giving you the ability to do the things you love without pain or injury. The fact that you picked up this book means you are interested in being able to garden pain free for life.

As function relates to purpose, sometimes as in gardening, we endure positions that exceed the tolerance for the body's tissues. The burden on these tissues results in pain signal from the body and the brain. We will show you how to build resilient tissues that will allow you to garden pain free for life. It is time to build strength, eliminate pain, and reduce your chance of injury through the movements of gardening. The next time you hear the word exercise you should think of the warm sun or the breeze on your face as you tend to your garden. Give us seven minutes and we will keep you gardening pain free for the rest of your life.

2 EAT

This book is about movement but it would be hard to justify writing a book about movement if we didn't touch on the importance of diet on overall well-being. Eating well is the foundation of health and without a proper diet you certainly will not be moving well. For those who are not eating well or are confused about what they should eat, this will be the most important part of this book.

What should we eat to be healthy? It seems like such a simple question doesn't it? So why then does it provoke the most complicated answers? This book aims to keep things simple and practical. Eating well can be broken down into three foundation principles that, if followed, will lead to a healthy and balanced diet.

When it comes to your diet, if you don't apply these principles, it really doesn't matter what diet plan or nutritional "expert" you are following, you are unlikely to find success. Not only will you continue to manipulate your body chemistry making each future attempt to lose weight more and more difficult, but you are going to waste your time doing it. The following principles will form your base of healthy eating and, by mastering them, you will be in a position to understand your diet, food, your body, and what works best for you. Your body will then be in a position to adopt new healthy changes to your diet on your terms. This is the key ingredient in creating new habits.

Principle One: Just Eat Real Food

As every gardener knows nothing tastes better than fresh food from your garden. I was introduced to the term JERF by a man named Sean Croxton who runs the website *Underground Wellness*. JERF means to Just Eat Real Food. While this principle may seem like common sense, it has been all but abandoned by many experts who push miracle products, elimination of entire foods groups, mailing pre-packaged food to you (this is just weird), and completely neglecting the quality of the food they are telling people to eat. As gardeners understand, there is a big difference in the quality of foods we see in pre-packaged meals and the ones we pull from our own garden, this principle will likely feel natural to you if you are used to growing your own food.

Before starting any healthy eating plan or "diet" you would be wise to make sure it takes into account the quality of the food you are putting into your body. In order to move, your body needs fuel and, without considering the quality of that fuel, you will be starting any diet from a faulty base. Might you lose weight from some wildly concocted diet or one that severely restricts your caloric intake? Sure. However, long term success isn't likely when we don't consider our body's needs or the quality of the food we choose to put into it. Many of you may have experienced the yo-yo like effect of these diets that promise rapid and permanent weight loss. The diet industry is a multi-billion dollar industry and it is only going to make money if you are not successful. If their diets worked, you wouldn't need to spend money on them anymore. They operate on the same principle as gambling. The first time you try it, you lose some weight, and then they know you will continue to spend money on diets hoping you will "win" again.

Although we have had clients try to convince us that rice crackers and honey nut cheerios are real food, we all know intuitively what real food is. Real food nourishes us and gives us energy. Real food grows from healthy soil or feeds on healthy plants. Real food we can grow ourselves and it generally isn't found in the frozen food isle. The problem with real food is that corporations cannot patent it and sell to you like they can their "proprietary products" although some are trying. Any so called nutritional "expert" that is not talking about real food and the quality of foods you are putting in your body is wasting your time. *Just Eat Real Food* and you will begin to see how much energy your body will have for daily movement; it will change your life forever.

Action Steps

1. Get to know your farmer and where your food comes from. Ask them questions and learn about the steps your farmer is taking to ensure you get real food on your table. A great place to get to know your farmer is at your local farmers market.

2. Start cooking. A sure fire way to know that your are just eating real food is by controlling the ingredients yourself. Make cooking a social event for your family or have friends over and have a real food potluck.

3. Plan your meals. There is nothing worse than ending your workday and not knowing what it is you are going to eat. Of course your are going to go for fast food. Plan a weeks worth of meals in advance, do your shopping, and stick to it.

4. Check out Real Food Friday on our Blog at www.sevenmovements.com where we will be sharing real food recipes perfect for you and your family every Friday.

Principle Two: Recognize that your optimal dietary requirements are unique

This is yet another simple principle that so many miss or choose to ignore. Your optimal dietary requirements are unique. There is no perfect diet that will fit every person on earth, period. We are all uniquely different on the inside just as we are on the outside. Why is this ignored? Promoters of diets won't tell people that their diet will only work with certain segments of the population; that would be cutting off a large portion of their possible market share. It is much easier to tell you they have a one sized fits all solution. This is simply not true. Understanding this principle will allow you to make sound personal decisions about your diet for the rest of your life. Without this understanding we can easily be sold on cheap quick fixes, get pulled into diet groups, and never understand why we are the only one not losing weight. If we do not recognize our uniqueness we will spend our lives following other people's diets instead of working to find our own personal optimal diet.

Our differences extend beyond our physical appearances. When the next celebrity comes out with a book or magazine article promoting a diet because it made them feel great we should not expect that it should do the same for us. In fact, we should understand it probably won't. Understanding this enables us to make better decisions about our diet choices. Empower yourself through the simple recognition that you are unique and need to find your own way. And to find your own way we must move on to principle three.

Action Steps

1. Throw away your magazines. Seriously, get rid of them. This way you won't be tempted when the next celebrity comes out with their own miracle diet. Nor will you be distracted by the next "study" that tells you that eating eggs are good for you followed by next weeks edition with a "study" that tells you eating eggs is bad for you. We have a list of recommended reading on our website if you wish to dive deeper into the subtleties of your diet.

2. Write these words down, " I am unique". Post them everywhere. Remind yourself constantly that you are a unique individual that will empower yourself through your own knowledge. Only you know what makes you feel best and don't forget it.

Principle Three: Learn to listen to your body

This principle is something that is going to help you drown out much of the noise coming from celebrities, nutritional "experts", and diet books. We often get it from all angles. Eat vegan! Eat Paleo! Follow Atkins! Follow South Beach! The list is endless. Experts, friends, and even family will often tell you that their way of eating is the only way that is good for you. By taking time to learn to listen to your body you will be able to know definitively whether or not what you are eating is working for you. You will know because you will connect how you feel to what you are eating. As trainers we have seen people on all types of diets from vegans to people following Atkins that made them feel tired and awful. On the flip side, we have had clients who moved to those same diets and it changed their lives for the better. This simply highlights how vital it is to learn to listen to your body as well as how unique the body is to each individual.

So many people are not only disconnected from the food they eat but from their own bodies as well. Lack of energy, indigestion, irritability, stress, soreness and so many more ailments are accepted as a normal part of life. It does not have to be this way, it is time to empower ourselves by learning to listen to our bodies. Our bodies have so much to tell us.

Your body will tell you which foods are giving you lasting energy and which are giving you a quick boost followed by a crash. It will tell you which foods make you feel tired and irritable and which foods give you a sense of strength and clarity. Many people will notice the obvious intolerances to food but many miss the subtleties. It is time to start really listening, if you are eating like your nutritional "expert" says you should and feel horrible, you need to listen to your body and try something else. Sometimes trial and error is the only way but remember you must also take into account principles one and two. Trust us, it will be worth it.

As you learn to listen to your body you will start to tune out all of the arguing going on between the diet experts and daily conflicting research because you will know what makes you feel at your best and what doesn't. When that friend drops by to tell you about his/her latest diet, you can smile and nod while knowing you are going to stick with what works for you. Embracing this principle will empower you to make decisions based on how food makes *you feel* rather than how someone else tells you it should make you feel.

Action Steps

1. Test test test. Recognize how you feel after you eat. Do you feel full? Do you feel hungry? Do you feel like napping? Full of energy? All of these symptoms could be a result of what you are eating.

2. If you have foods you suspect are bothering your digestion or making you feel poorly start by eliminating them for two weeks at a time. Do you feel a difference?

3. Bring some variety into your diet. Stagger the types of foods you are eating and you will be able to recognize the subtleties of how certain types of foods are making you feel.

The purpose of this book is to inspire you to move. When you learn to eat right you have the energy and capacity to move how you want to. Allow these principles to be your measuring stick before attempting any diet plan. It is important to remember that there are many excellent nutritional experts out there that are ready to guide you through this process should you require it, but be sure their practices are rooted in the foundation that these principles represent as they are unchanging. We hope you can take them and free yourself to make the choices you need to make to feel better and live healthier. Good luck and happy eating!

3 MOVE

Movement is life. In this section of the book we are going to give you seven simple movements that will help you to continue gardening for life. They are going to help you avoid injury, keep your joints healthy, and change the way you view the word "exercise" forever. When speaking with gardeners, we often hear complaints of aching joints and sore backs. As personal trainers there is nothing that pains us more than seeing someone lose the ability to move whether it be due to age or injury. Know that it does not have to be this way.

Movement need not be complicated to be effective. The exercise industry has done a terrible job of promoting this concept. Our bodies have been designed to move from the beginning of time. In the diet section of this book, we talked about recognizing our individuality and now we need to realize that our movements might also need to be unique. The way we get around the garden might look very different from our neighbor and that's ok. We are going to look at the very fundamentals of what keeps our bodies moving successfully (meaning without pain). We want to give you simple tools to enjoy the movement you express daily in your gardens.

Some gardeners would spend their entire day in their garden if they could. The problem is some activities involved in gardening include holding ourselves in a static position over a long period of time whether it be kneeling, squatting, or standing up bent over our plants. This lends itself to pain and stiffness in the joints which can lead to injury. We have designed seven movements that will combat some of the common injuries and pains that can creep into our bodies from prolonged bouts of gardening by hydrating and strengthening your connective tissue allowing you to keep gardening for life.

These seven simple movements will help you gain the freedom to keep gardening on your terms. When you enter your garden you are, in fact, exercising. Not everyone enjoys the gym and you don't need to spend time in a gym to enjoy movement. Allow your passions to guide you to a stronger and healthier body that will keep you moving for life.

Allow us to guide you through these movements, perform them together in one seven minute warm up prior to getting into the garden or perform them individually before performing certain gardening movements.

1.   Weeding

We start with the most frustrating chore in gardening. Weeding, although annoying, is an integral process for the growth and development of our plants and food. We want all the nutrients and water to get to the plants. Without weeding the nutrients in the soil would struggle to gain access to our vegetables or flowers. The skill of weeding involves a variety of positions. Those positions may include being bent over, squatting, seated and probably kneeling. We may also be standing using a weeding tool.

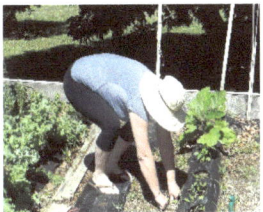

Prolonged time spent in any static position is detrimental to the health of your body, specifically your connective tissue (muscles, fascia, tendons, ligaments, skin). Let's get moving to help prevent this damage.

Bend

If you are someone that spends a great deal of time weeding your garden, let us show you a movement that you can do that will enhance your ability to weed for a sustained period of time. without pain or injury.

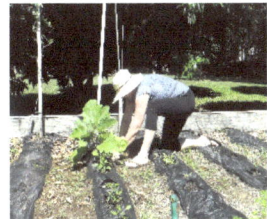

Half Kneel

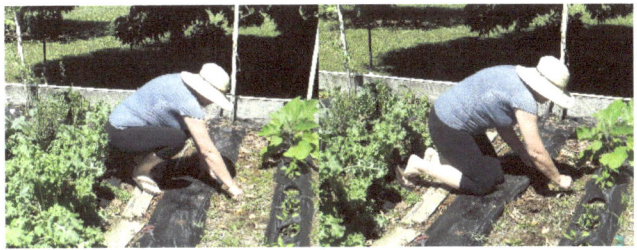

Squat/Kneel

The goal of this enhancer is to create extension in the middle of your back! This is the counteracting motion of that sustained weeding posture. We are unloading the thoracic spine into an extended position and out of the bent or flexed (rounded) position of the back. This will enhance your body's ability to weed for longer periods of time.

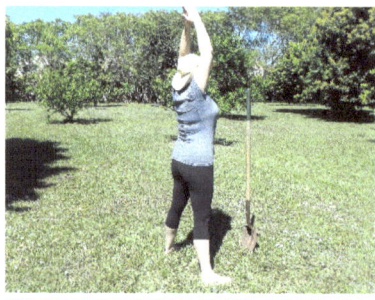

- Stand and extend arms above head

- Keep spine tall

- Pull Spine upwards to keep it tall
- Extend arms and grab shovel

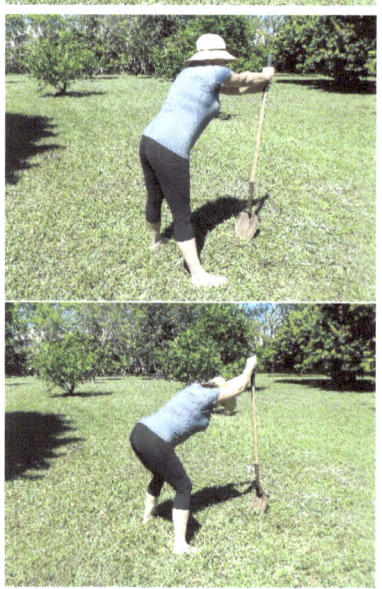

- Reach from your shoulder blades

- Move from the hips and pelvis

- Push hips back

Perform this movement for 1 minute prior to weeding and for 1 minute for every seven minutes of weeding!

2. Planting

Working in the garden is such a delightful activity. Especially when it comes to making the decision of what you are going to plant. Once you choose those special seeds it is time to work the soil and plant them in the ground. We have several positions we may plant in.

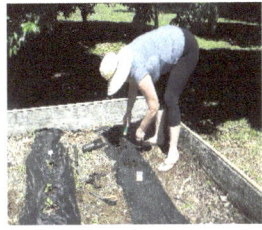

The bent over position or forward flexed position is very common. We introduce the seated position and the kneeling position too. It is important to vary your positioning to keep the body's connective tissues hydrated and resilient for the chores of gardening. As usual movement is key.

Bend

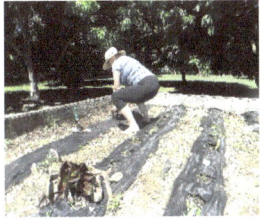

Let us show you a simple movement that you can perform prior to planting to enhance the body's ability to plant for a sustained amount of time without pain and/or injury

Squat

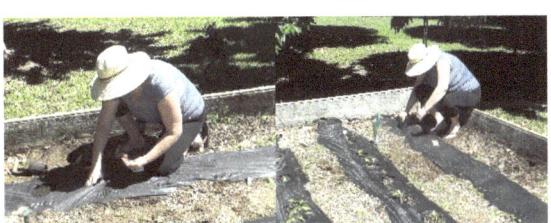

Kneel/Seated

The goal of this enhancer is to lengthen the muscles in the front of the hip and pull the spine tall! This will help you combat those aches and pains you might feel after a long planting session.

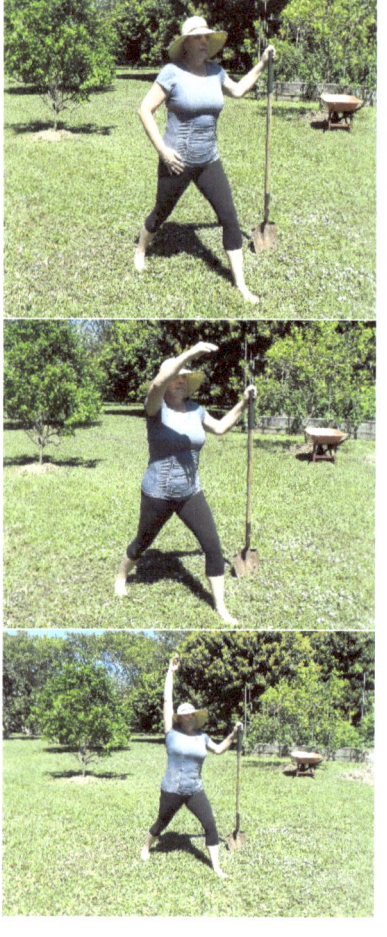

- In a split stance pull your spine upwards to keep it as tall as you can

- Reach to the sky with your opposite arm

- Reach from your shoulder blades

- Move from the hips and pelvis

- Slowly move front hips forward into a stretch

Perform this movement prior to planting for one minute. You can also perform this movement when you start to feel like you are stiffening up during planting.

3.   Shoveling

Shoveling can be some gardeners most hated chore. Allow us to make it your favorite. The shoveling movement can be broken into 3 separate motions. Shoveling begins as a step and bend (placing the shovel in the manure) squat and lift (lifting the manure) and rotate and shift (emptying the shovel). This motion is extremely difficult for those that suffer from back pain.

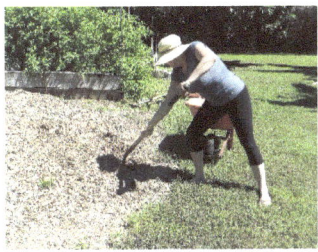

In order to be successful (pain free) with this movement we need to create extension and rotation to protect the spine from its most vulnerable position. The position to avoid when shoveling is forward bending while side bending.

Step & Bend

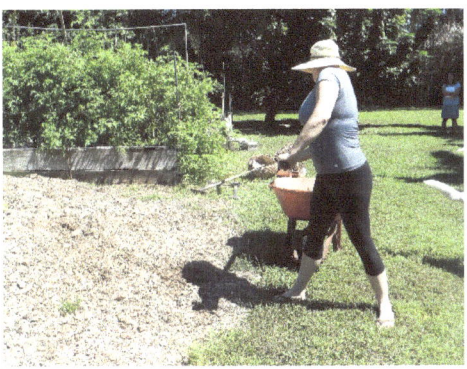

Rotate & Shift

Let us show you the simple movement you can perform to enhance your body's ability to avoid injuries and pain while shoveling.

The goal of this enhancer is to create extension in the spine and rotation in the hips and spine. This will help you avoid common injuries and pain many associate with shoveling.

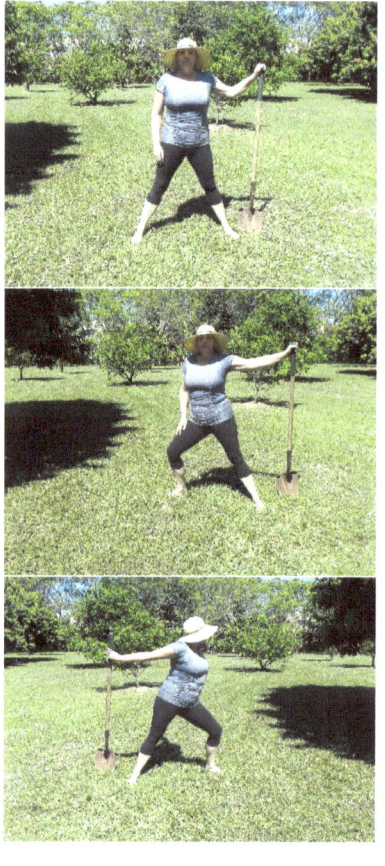

- Begin with a wide stance

- Slowly move hips away from shovel while keeping spine tall

- Keeping your arm on the tool rotate your hips away from the tool

- Reach and extend arm away from the body

Perform this movement for 1 minute prior to shoveling.

4. Digging

Digging as we describe it is a much different movement than shoveling. There are times when we need to dig holes to plant shrubs, trees or even turn up potatoes. Digging can be a struggle especially if you have tough soil and rocks in the way.

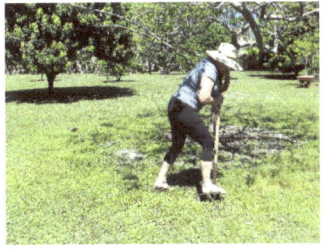

This can lead to annoying aches and pains and an all around negative perception of digging. Allow us to change that perception and prepare you body for this movement.

Step/Plunge

There are three parts to the Digging movement. They are Step or Plunge, Pry or Pull, and Lift.

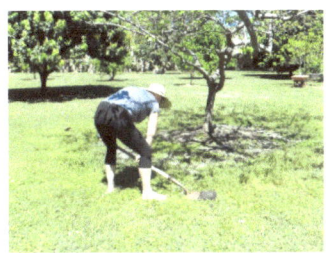

Pry/Pull

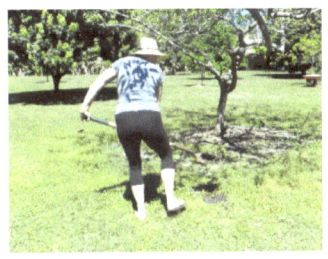

Let us show you a simple movement that will help enhance your body's ability to dig for an extended period of time without those dreaded aches and pains.

Lift

The goal of this enhancer is to create mobility in the ankle hip and spine. We inherently have more stability if we have more mobility in the joints. By increasing mobility we will create greater spaces between joint surfaces and relieve joint pain.

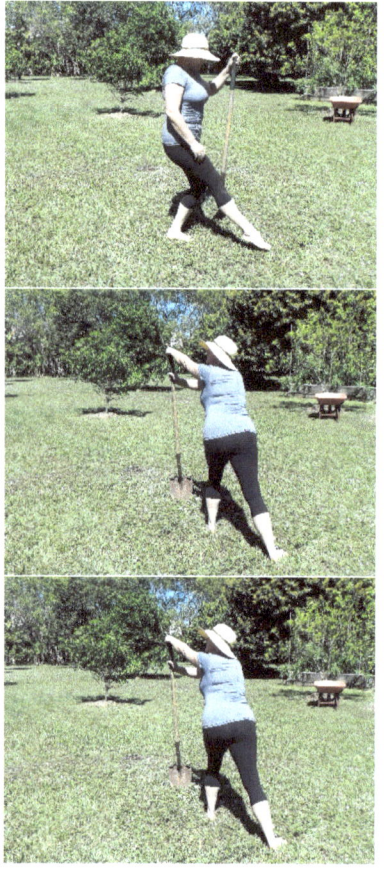

- Put all weight onto one leg (use tool for balance

- Extend opposite leg towards ground

- Take step back with elevated leg and grab tool with opposite hand

- Rotate body inward towards tool while keeping spine tall

Perform this movement for 1 minute prior to digging.

5. Raking or hoeing

Some consider raking or hoeing a serene relaxing task, others who are experiencing pain dread even the site of a rake. Raking involves both a reaching and pulling motion which can result in pain if the body is not prepared for this motion.

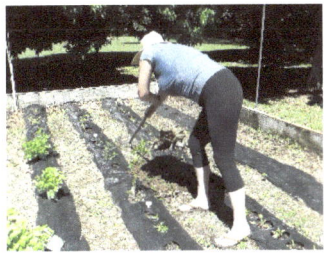

However, this movement can also be an effective exercise. Allow us to show you how to rake more effectively allowing it to become the relaxing task it is meant to be.

Reach

Let us show you a simple movement to enhance your bodies ability to rake effectively and without pain.

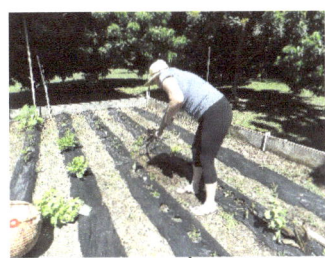 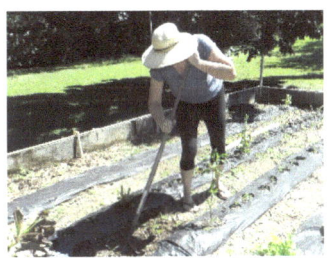

Pushing /Pulling

The goal of this Raking enhancer is to mobilize the lateral side of the body. This will allow the shoulders to glide along the rib cage and make reaching and dragging the rake/ hoe through the soil more efficient.

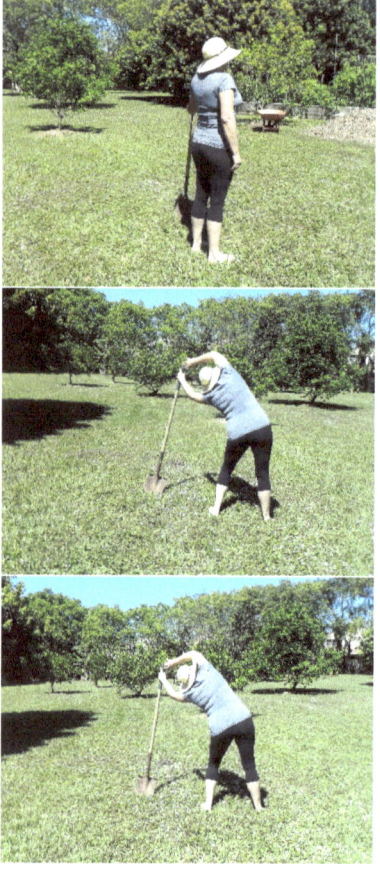

- Stand with a shoulder width stance

- Move hips to side away from tool

- Reach overhead and push hips in opposite direction of tool

Perform this movement for 30 seconds on each side prior to raking.

6. Transport - Drag, Carry, Dump

Dragging, Carrying and Dumping and Wheel barrel are considered what we call loaded movement exercises. It consists of a specific movement while under load. In this case we are relocating fertilizer or soil.

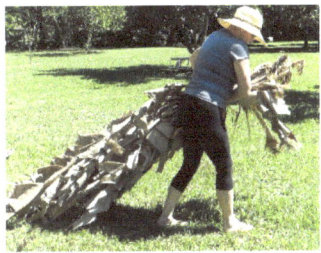

This can be a very strenuous task and lead to significant injuries. Because this type of exercise requires the entire body we will prepare the entire body with these movement enhancers.

Drag

Let us show you a simple movement you can perform to enhance your body's ability to handle these types of loaded movements.

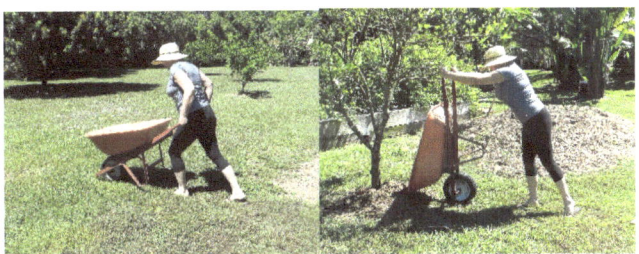

Carry/Dump

The goal of the transport enhancer is to prepare the entire body to have the ability to stiffen when moving with a load. In order to provide tension through the body to stabilize a load outside of the body we must be able to move freely in the ankles, hips and mid back. This one movement is the Swiss Army Knife of movement enhancers! It does it all!

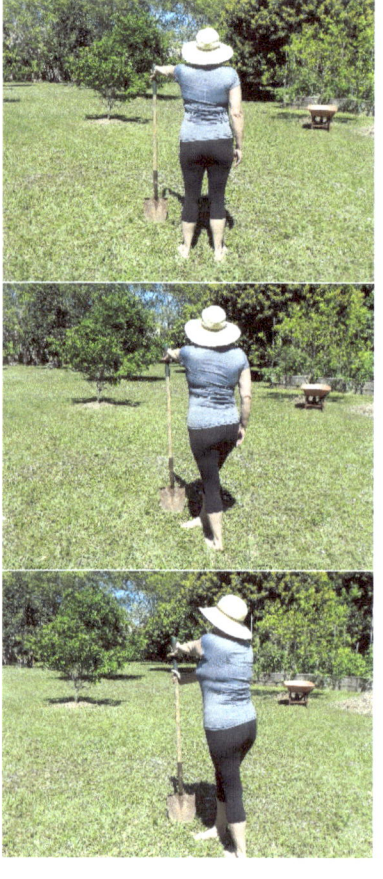

- Put left hand on top of the shovel, thumb turned down

- Put right foot forward and turn inward to 9 o'clock

- Then turn same foot outward to 4'oclock

- Turn head to follow path of the foot

Perform this movement for 1 minute prior to transporting anything in your garden.

7. Lift

The lift movement can be described as moving an object from a low position on earth to a higher position. We all know the subsequent injuries that can take place when our body is not prepared to lift. We can lift objects with our hands or other parts of the body as well as move objects with tools. It is important to vary the direction you are lifting objects and over different distances and heights.

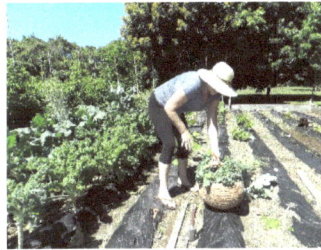

Bend

It is also healthy to change the position of your feet and hands relative to the object you are lifting. The tissues become stronger, more resilient, and will have more energy stored in them. Thus allowing you to garden for a longer period of time.

Let us show you a simple movement you can perform to enhance your body's ability to perform a lifting movement.

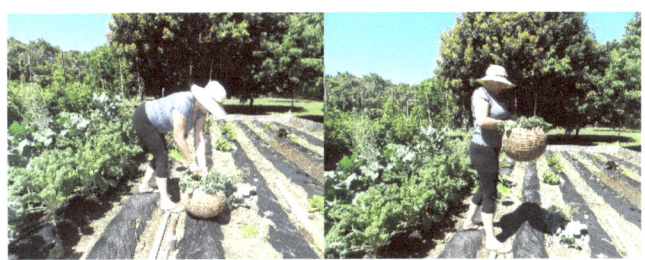

Reach/Lift

The goal of the lift enhancer is to lengthen the tissues around the pelvis and the arms. The wider stance and shifting of your hips will allow the pelvis to open up. This will help you reach lower and bend lower to pick up heavier objects in lower positions.

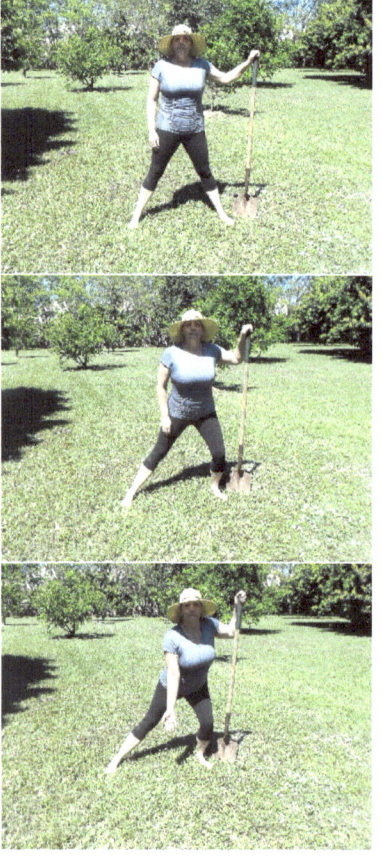

- Place feet in wide stance

- Shift weight towards tool

- Push hips back

- Reach opposite hand towards ground

Perform this movement for 1 minute prior to lifting and remember to move slowly. Your tissues will thank you.

Thank you so much for being a part of Seven Movements.

For more information on new books, apps, and other free goodies please visit us at:

www.sevenmovements.com

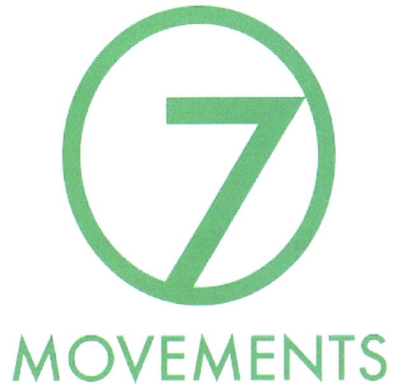

ABOUT THE AUTHORS

John Sinclair

When Dan Tatton asked me to collaborate on this project I could not have been more excited. We both realized that the fitness industry was moving in the opposite direction of where we are needed most. While other personal trainers search for the newest and craziest exercises, Dan and I noticed that we need to share the simplest and most effective movements to help people enjoy the activities that they are currently doing. It was becoming ridiculous to me that my clients were joining a gym just to regain strength and stamina to be able to do the things they loved to do outside of the gym.

In an effort to help people deal with their complaints we created this book to provide solutions to your problems. These problems may include back and joint pain, chronic headaches, fibromyalgia and other musculoskeletal disorders. We want you to have the ability to do what you love, when you want to do it and for as long as possible. These movements that we have created for you are simple, replicable and most importantly they work!

I would be remiss if I didn't thank my mentors and friends. The people that helped me become the coach I am today. My friend and former General Manager Jeff Thirsk, you have always supported me in any endeavor I have taken on. Michol Dalcourt, Scott Hopson, Rodney Corn, Bobby Cappuccio, Richard Boyd, and the entire faculty of PTA Global and Institute of Motion. A special thanks to Ian ODwyer who has helped me simplify movement and has inspired me to include his concept of Mobilizers into this book. You the reader will experience life changing movement with the Enhancers we have included in this book. Check out our app so you can see how we have expanded the book into coaching sessions. This will really bring the book to life.

Good luck and happy gardening.

Dan Tatton

Partnering with John Sinclair on this book has been an incredible experience. As personal trainers we want the world to experience more movement. Movement is life and when we experience it free of pain and with strength we feel connected to our bodies. We have been given the gift of choosing how we want to experience movement on a daily basis. Let's take advantage of that and do what we love to do.

This book is an effort to give you the simplest most effective tools you need to experience successful movement in the garden. It aims to flip the " no pain, no gain" attitude on its head and allow you to build strength, eliminate pain, and begin moving with ease.

The reason I started writing this book was to help those that want to find health. It is a guide that aims to give you the simplest tools you need to experience movement in a positive way. It is to help those that don't enjoy going into a gym or pushing themselves to exhaustion to achieve what the industry tells us is success. It is for those that simply want to do what they love to do for as long as they possibly can free from pain and discomfort.

Three years ago I set out to create an exercise program that was connected to your passion, easy and convenient to do, and supplemented the movement you already love to do. John was the perfect partner as he is the most brilliant movement specialist I have had the honor of seeing in action. Together, I knew we could change the way people look at exercise forever.

Writing this book has been a dream come true for me and I would like to thank all those that helped make it a reality. There are too many to list but you know who you are and all of you inspire me everyday.